Air Fryer Cookbook
Side Dishes
&
Dinner

40+ Air Fryer Dinner Recipes with Low Salt, Low Fat and Less Oil.

The Healthier Way to Enjoy Deep-Fried Flavours

Ronda Williams

Table of Contents

Introduction

What is Air Frying?

First, a quick explanation of what air frying is and isn't. They don't fry food at all. They are more like a self-contained convection oven than a deep fat fryer. Most units have one or more heating elements, along with a fan or two to circulate the hot air. These appliances quickly heat and circulate the hot air around and through the food in the tray. This cooking method takes advantage of the heat and the drying effect of the air to cook foods quickly, leaving them crisp and browned on the outside but still moist inside. While the results can be similar to using a deep fryer, they are not identical.

What Are The Pros And Cons Of An Air Fryer?

While the enthusiasm about these products may be a bit overblown, there are some solid benefits to using an air fryer, as well as some major downsides.

Pros Of An Air Fryer

1. Healthier Meals

You do not need to use much (or any) oil in these appliances to get your food crispy and browned! Most users just spritz a little oil on the item and then proceed to the cooking cycle. The hot air takes advantage of the little bit of oil, and any excess oil just drains away from the food. This makes these devices ideal for making fresh and frozen fries, onion rings, mozzarella sticks, chicken wings, and nuggets. Unlike a traditional oven, air frying items are cooked faster and the excess oil doesn't soak into your food. So the claims that they use less oil and make healthier meals are true!

2. Quicker, More Efficient Cooking

Air fryers take just minutes to preheat, and most of the heat stays inside the appliance. Foods cook faster than in an oven or on a stovetop because this heat is not lost to the surrounding air. Even frozen foods are quickly cooked because the effect of the heat is intensified by the circulating air. These units are also more energy-efficient than an oven. Using a fryer will not heat your house in the summer, and the cost of the electricity used is just pennies. Since the cooking cycle is also shorter, you can see that using a fryer makes most cooking faster and more efficient than traditional appliances!

3. Versatility

You can use them to air fry, stir fry, reheat, bake, broil, roast, grill, steam, and even rotisserie in some models. Besides the fries and nuggets, you can make hot dogs and sausages, steak, chicken breasts or thighs, grilled sandwiches, stir-fried meats and veggies, roasted or steamed veggies, all kinds of fish and shrimp dishes, even cakes and desserts. If your unit is large enough, you can even bake a whole chicken or small turkey, or do a beef or pork roast. They are more than just a fryer!

4. Space-Saving

Most units are about the size of a coffee maker. Some models are small and super-compact, making them perfect for small kitchens, kitchenettes, dorm rooms, or RVs. An air fryer can replace an oven in a situation that lacks one and can be more useful than a toaster oven or steamer. If you use it frequently you will likely be happy to give it a home on your kitchen counter!

5. Easy To Use

Most fryers are designed to be easy to use. Just set the cooking temperature and time, put your food in the basket, and walk away. Of course, you will get better results if you shake your food once or twice during the cooking cycle, especially for things like fries, chips, wings, and nuggets. This ensures even browning and perfect results. Many air fryer enthusiasts have even taught their children to use them for making after school snacks or quick lunches!

Cons of an Air Fryer

1. Quality Issues

Air fryers are mostly made from plastic and inexpensive metal parts. They may or may not bear up after months or years of use. The heating elements, controls, and fans tend to go out eventually, and once they do your unit is useless. The metal cooking baskets and pans do not tend to last very long and often need to be replaced. Print on the dials or control panels can wear off. Even expensive units can have these issues, and some brands seem to have a lot of reported problems. These are not sturdy, long-lasting kitchen appliances overall.

2. Takes Up Space

Ok, I had "Space Saver" listed as a pro...how can it be a con as well? Easy! They do take up space, either on your counter or stored away in a cabinet. If you use it frequently this might not be a problem...but if you only drag it out to make the occasional batch of wings then the loss of space might not make it worth it to you. It depends on how and if you use it. Some units are fairly heavy as well, and might not be very easy to move around. They have the potential to be just another appliance you use a few times and then sell at a yard sale.

3. Not Ideal For Large Families

You will see some fryers advertised for "large families" but what does that mean? Most air fryers are best suited to making food for 1-4 people (depending on the capacity). There are very few that can handle making food for more than 4, and they often still require cooking in batches. For large families, a true convection air frying oven would probably be a better choice.

A medium-sized fryer with a capacity of 3.5 quarts can usually handle the main dish for two or a main and side dish for one. A large unit with a capacity of 5.8 quarts can handle the main dish like a whole chicken...which theoretically means enough to serve 4 people, as long as you cook the rest of the food in another appliance. So these are ideal for smaller families or single users, or a dorm or office snack maker.

4. Learning Curve

They ARE easy to use, but there is still a learning curve. Each unit has its peculiarities that you will have to figure out. They come with cooking guides and recipes, but those are more recommendations rather than firm instructions. It may take a few trials before you get the results that you want. Luckily the internet is filled with users who have shared their experiences, so finding tips is pretty easy.

5. Limitations

For all their versatility, air fryers have limitations as well. You are limited by the size and shape of the basket. Your frozen taquitos may not fit into some models, and you might be limited to a 6-inch pie pan in another. Food sometimes gets stuck to the cooking pans, meaning a more difficult clean-up for you. Even with accessories like elevated cooking racks and kabob skewers, you will still have to cook in batches or use another appliance if you are making food for multiple people.

You also have to wait for the unit to cool off before cleaning and storing it away. For some people, these limitations might be too much to make an air fryer worth it.

Air Fryer Benefits

- An air fryer has many benefits to offer its customers.
- Low-fat meals
- Easy cleanup
- Uses hot-air circulation, the air fryer cooks your ingredients from all angles- with no oil needed.
- This ultimately produces healthier foods than most fryers and spares you from that unwanted aroma of fried foods in your home.
- To make sure you get the most out of your appliance, most fryers are accompanied by a recipe book to help you get started right away on your journey of fast, yet healthy meal preparations.
- Whether your favorite dish is french fries, muffins, chips, chicken tenders, or grilled vegetables, an air fryer can prepare it all.

Is an Air Fryer Useful?

At the tip of your fingers, you can have an appliance that specializes in making delicious, healthy meals that look and taste just like the ones made in oil fryers. The air fryer serves up many ways to be useful in your life.

Consider:

- Do you find yourself short on time to cook?
- Are you having a hard time letting go of those fatty foods, but still want to lose weight?
- Are you always seeking to get a bang for your buck?

If you answered yes to any of these questions, then an air fryer may be for you.

Why You Should Use An Air Fryer

An air fryer can pretty much do it all. And by all, we mean fry, grill, bake, and roast. Equipped with sturdy plastic and metal material, the air fryer has many great benefits to offer.

Air Fryers Can:

- Cook multiple dishes at once
- Cut back on fatty oils
- Prepare a meal within minutes
- While every appliance has its cons, the air fryer doesn't offer many.
- The fryer may be bulky in weight, but its dimensions are slimmer than most fryers. An air fryer can barely take up any counter space.
- If you need fast, healthy, convenient, and tasty, then once again, an air fryer may be for you.

Air Fryer- Healthier

The biggest quality the air fryer offers is healthier dishes

In comparison to other fryers, air fryers were designed to specifically function without fattening oils and to produce food with up to 80 percent less fat than food cooked with other fryers. The air fryer can help you lose the weight, you've been dying to get rid of. While it can be difficult to let go of your favorite fried foods, an air fryer will let you have your cake and eat it too. You can still have your fried dishes, but at the same time, still conserve those calories and saturated fat. The air fryer can also grill, bake, and roast foods as well. Offering you an all in one combination, the air fryer is the perfect appliance for anyone looking to switch to a healthier lifestyle.

Fast And Quick

- If you're on a tight schedule, you may want to use an air fryer.
- Within minutes you can have crunchy golden fries or crispy chicken tenders.
- This fryer is perfect for people who are constantly on the go and do not have much time to prepare meals.
- With most air fryers, french fries can be prepared within 12 minutes.
- That cuts the time you spend in the kitchen by a tremendous amount.

Features

1. Temperature And Timer

- Avoid the waiting time for your fryer to decide when it wants to heat up.
- With an air fryer, once you power it on, the fryer will instantly heat.
- When using the appliance cold, that is, right after it has been off for a while (since last use) all you have to do is add three minutes to your cooking time to allow for it to heat up properly.
- The appliance is equipped with adjustable temperature control that allows you to set the temperature that can be altered for each of your meals.
- Most fryers can go up to 200-300 degrees.
- Because the fryer can cook food at record times, it comes with a timer that can be pre-set with no more than 30 minutes.
- You can even check on the progress of your foods without messing up the set time. Simply pull out the pan, and the fryer will cause heating. When you replace the pan, heating will resume.
- When your meal is prepared and your timer runs out, the fryer

will alert you with its ready sound indicator. But just in-case you can't make it to the fryer when the timer goes, the fryer will automatically switch off to help prevent your ingredients from overcooking and burning.

2. Food Separator

Some air fryers are supplied with a food separator that enables you to prepare multiple meals at once. For example, if you wanted to prepare frozen chicken nuggets and french fries, you could use the separator to cook both ingredients at the same time, all the while avoiding the worry of the flavors mixing. An air fryer is perfect for quick and easy, lunch and dinner combinations. It is recommended to pair similar ingredients together when using the separator. This will allow both foods to share a similar temperature setting.

3. Air Filter

Some air fryers are built with an integrated air filter that eliminates those unwanted vapors and food odors from spreading around your house. No more smelling like your favorite fried foods, the air filter will diffuse that hot oil steam that floats and sticks. You can now enjoy your fresh kitchen smell before, during, and after using your air fryer.

4. Cleaning

- No need to fret after using an air fryer, it was designed for hassle-free cleaning.
- The parts of the fryer are constructed of non-stick material.
- This prevents any food from sticking to surfaces that ultimately make it hard to clean.
- It is recommended to soak the parts of the appliances before cleaning.
- All parts such as the grill, pan, and basket are removable and dishwasher friendly.

- After your ingredients are cooked to perfection, you can simply place your parts in the dishwasher for a quick and easy clean.

Tips on Cleaning an Air Fryer:

- Use detergent that specializes in dissolving oil.
- For a maximum and quick cleaning, leave the pan to soak in water and detergent for a few minutes.
- Avoid using metal utensils when cleaning the appliance to prevent scuffs and scratches on the material.
- Always let the fryer cool off for about 30 minutes before you wash it.

5. Cost-effective

Are there any cost-effective air fryers? For all that they can do, air fryers can be worth the cost. It has been highly questionable if the benefits of an air fryer are worth the expense. When you weigh your pros and cons, the air fryer surely leads with its pros. There aren't many fryers on the market that can fry, bake, grill and roast; and also promise you healthier meals. An air fryer saves you time, and could potentially save you money. Whether the air fryer is cost-effective for your life, is ultimately up to you.

The air fryer is a highly recommendable appliance to anyone starting a new diet, parents with busy schedules, or individuals who are always on the go. Deciding whether the investment is worth it, is all up to the purchaser. By weighing the air fryer advantages and the unique differences the air fryer has, compared to other fryers, you should be able to decide whether the air fryer has a lot to bring to the table.

Recipes

1. <u>Air Fryer Broccoli Cheese Bites</u>

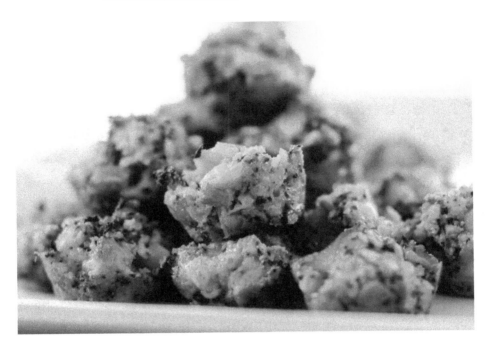

Prep Time: 50 mins

Active Time: 20 mins

Total Time: 1 hr 10 mins

Ingredients

- 10 oz. fresh broccoli florets
- 1/4 cup water
- 1 large egg
- 1 1/2 cups shredded cheddar cheese
- 3/4 cup bread crumbs (panko or traditional)
- 1/2 tsp. kosher salt

- 1/2 tsp. black pepper

Instructions

- Place broccoli and water in a microwave-safe container with a microwave-safe lid (if you don't have a lid you can use plastic wrap). Place lid lightly on top or cover tightly with plastic wrap. Microwave for 4 minutes.
- Remove from microwave and allow to cool enough to handle. Chop very finely then place in a bowl. Add egg, cheese, bread crumbs, salt, and pepper to the broccoli and mix well. Grab a rimmed baking sheet.
- Scoop out 1 1/2 tablespoons of the broccoli mixture and squeeze and form into a ball. Set on a baking sheet. Continue until you've used all the mixture. Place in the freezer for 30 minutes.
- Place broccoli bites in an air fryer in a single layer and cook at 350 degrees F for 5-10 minutes depending on your air fryer. You may need to do this in batches (I did). Cover lightly with foil to keep warm while others are baking.

Nutritional Facts

- Calories: 91kcal | Carbohydrates: 6g | Protein: 2g | Fat: 7g | Saturated Fat: 1g | Sodium: 300mg | Potassium: 296mg | Fiber: 1g | Sugar: 4g | Vitamin A: 196IU | Vitamin C: 20mg | Calcium: 25mg | Iron: 1mg

2. Healthy Air Fryer Eggplant [Oil Free]

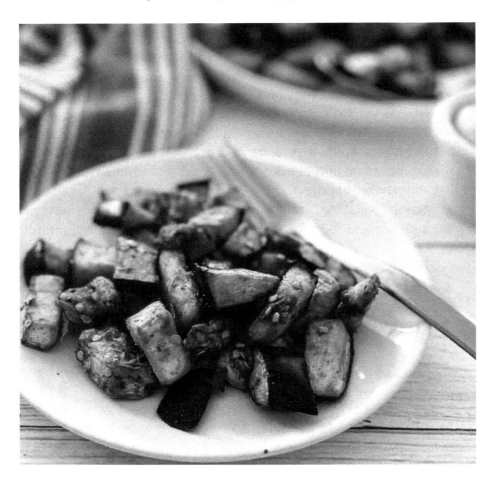

Prep Time: 35 minutes

Cook Time: 15 minutes

Total Time: 50 minutes

Ingredients

- 1.5 lb eggplant cut into half-inch pieces (approx 1 medium-sized)

- 2 tbsp low sodium vegetable broth
- 1 tsp garlic powder
- 1 tsp paprika
- 1/2 tsp dried oregano
- 1/4 tsp dried thyme
- 1/4 tsp black pepper optional

Instructions

- Wash and dice your eggplant into half-inch pieces. (See step by step photos above if needed.)
- Now place your cut up eggplant in a large colander and place the colander inside a bowl. Generously sprinkle with salt and let it sit for 30 minutes. Then transfer to a clean, dry dishtowel, and using another dish towel, or paper towels, press and pat them dry.
- Now, wipe out the bowl that was sitting under your colander and place the dry eggplant inside. Add the broth and all the seasoning to the bowl and mix well to evenly coat the pieces.
- Place in your air fryer basket, set to 380 degrees, and cook for 15-20 minutes, tossing once at the halfway point. Cook until nicely golden, and fork-tender, then serve warm with a sprinkle of fresh parsley or chives and sriracha mayo for dipping.

Nutrition Facts

- Calories: 48kcal | Carbohydrates: 11g | Protein: 2g | Fat: 1g | Saturated Fat: 1g | Sodium: 161mg | Potassium: 413mg | Fiber: 5g | Sugar: 6g | Vitamin A: 322IU | Vitamin C: 4mg | Calcium: 15mg | Iron: 1mg

3. <u>Air Fryer Tortilla Chips</u>

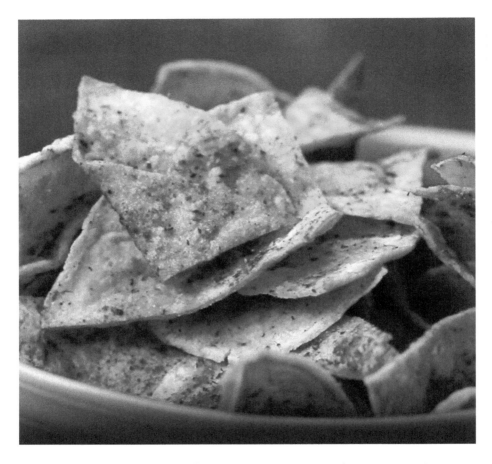

Prep Time: 10 minutes Cook Time: 9 minutes Total Time: 19 minutes

Ingredients

Salt And Vinegar

- 6 corn tortillas
- 1 tablespoon extra virgin olive oil
- 1/2 tablespoon white vinegar
- 1 teaspoon kosher salt

Zesty Cheese

- 6 corn tortillas
- 2 tablespoons extra virgin olive oil
- 2 teaspoons **Nutrition Facts**al yeast
- 1/2 teaspoon smoked paprika
- 1/4 teaspoon kosher salt

Spicy Chipotle

- 6 corn tortillas
- 1 tablespoon extra virgin olive oil
- 1/2 teaspoon ground chipotle chili pepper
- 1/4 teaspoon kosher salt

Chili Lime

- 6 corn tortillas
- 1 tablespoon extra virgin olive oil
- 1/2 tablespoon lime juice
- 1 teaspoon chili powder
- 1/4 teaspoon kosher salt

Maple Cinnamon

- 6 corn tortillas
- 1 tablespoon extra virgin olive oil
- 1/2 tablespoon maple syrup
- 1/2 teaspoon ground cinnamon
- 1/2 teaspoon coconut sugar

Instructions

- In a small bowl, whisk together the oil with the ingredients for your flavor choice. Brush a light coating of the mixture on both sides of the tortillas.
- Cut each tortilla into quarters to form triangles.

- Arrange the tortilla triangles in a single layer in your air fryer basket. (You will need to do this in batches).
- Air fry on 350F for about 7-9 minutes, or until they start to brown around the edges. (Note: the maple cinnamon chips will take 5-7 minutes).
- Let the chips cool enough to handle and then transfer them to a wire rack to cool completely. They will get crunchier as they cool.
- Store in an airtight container at room temperature and enjoy within 5 days.

Nutritional Facts

- Calories: 156
- Total Fat: 6g
- Total Carbohydrate: 24g
- Sugar: 0g
- Calcium: 91.6mg
- Sat Fat: 0.8g
- Sodium: 780.9mg
- Fiber: 2.7g
- Protein: 3g

4. **Air Fryer Asparagus**

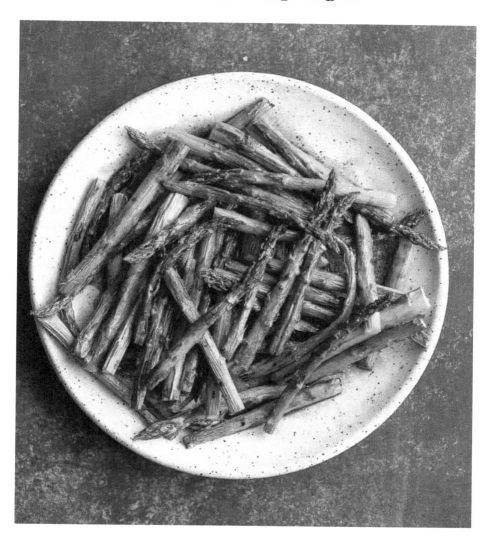

Prep Time: 5 minutes

Cook Time: 6 minutes

Total Time: 11 minutes

Ingredients

- 1 lb fresh asparagus (16 oz.)
- 2 tsp extra virgin olive oil
- Sea salt to taste

Instructions

- Wash the asparagus spears and pat them dry. Trim the ends enough so that they fit in the air fryer basket (about 1 to 1 ½ inches up from the bottom).
- Add the asparagus to a rectangular container with a tight-fitting lid or a zip-top bag along with the olive oil and salt. Shake until asparagus is well-coated.
- If your air fryer has a separate elevated crisping tray or plate, be sure to insert it. Add the asparagus to the air fryer basket and air fry at 400° F for 6-9 minutes, shaking the basket every few minutes. Thinner spears will take less time to cook while thicker spears will take longer. Asparagus should be tender with a slight crisp. Add more sea salt to taste before serving, if desired.

Nutrition

- Calories: 43kcal | Carbohydrates: 4g | Protein: 2g | Fat: 2g | Saturated Fat: 1g | Fiber: 2g

5. Air Fryer Pumpkin Fries

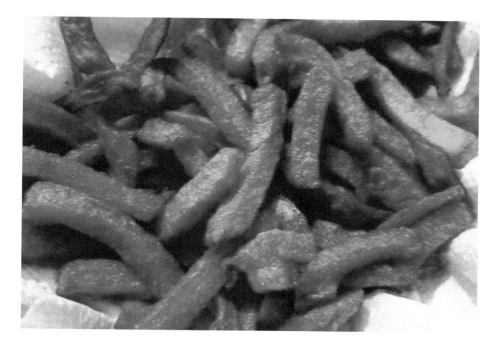

Prep Time: 15 minutes Cook Time: 15 minutes Total Time: 30 minutes

Ingredients

- 2 mini pumpkins, peeled, seeded, and cut into 1/2-inch slices (see cutting tips above)
- 2 teaspoons extra virgin olive oil
- 1/2 teaspoon garlic powder
- 1/2 teaspoon smoked paprika
- 1/2 teaspoon kosher salt

Instructions

- Quicker version – air fry in one large batch:
- Add the pumpkin slices to a large bowl and toss with oil and seasonings.
- Place all the pumpkin in the air fryer basket and air fry on 400F

for about 15 minutes, or until fork-tender. Shake or stir them at the mid-way point.

Nutritional Facts

- Calories: 60
- Total Fat: 2.5g
- Total Carbohydrate: 10g
- Sugar: 4g
- Calcium: 31.4mg
- Sat Fat: 0.4g
- Sodium: 156.9mg
- Fiber: 0.9g
- Protein: 1.6g
- Vitamin C: 13.1mg
- Iron: 1.2mg

6. <u>Lemon Garlic Air Fryer Roasted Potatoes</u>

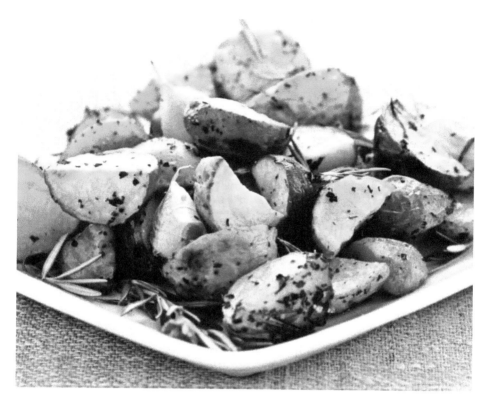

Prep Time: 10 Mins

Cook Time: 30 Mins

Air Fryer Preheating Time: 5 Mins

Total Time: 45 Mins

Ingredients

- 900 g / 2 lb potatoes (about 4 large ones)
- 2 tablespoons oil of choice, avocado, olive, vegetable, sunflower are all fine
- 1 teaspoon salt

25

- 1 teaspoon freshly ground black pepper
- 2 lemons
- 1 entire head of garlic
- 4 big (approx 4 inches long) fresh rosemary stems
- Peel the potatoes and cut them into large pieces. With a large potato, I generally get 5 pieces.
- Put the cut potatoes in a bowl and cover with cold water. Leave to soak for 15 minutes, then drain and pour the potatoes onto a clean dish towel. Bundle it up around them and rub them dry.
- Dry the bowl you had them in and return them, then pour in the oil and sprinkle in the salt and pepper. Stir to coat them all evenly.
- Preheat your Air Fryer if it has a preheat function, then add the potatoes carefully to the hot basket and cook on 350°F (175 °C) for 15 minutes.
- While they are cooking, break up the head of garlic into individual cloves and remove any skin that is loose and papery. Leave the rest of the skin intact.
- Cut the 2 lemons in half lengthways. Save one half for juicing, then cut the other halves into 3 wedges each.
- Once the 15 minutes is up, open the Air Fryer and squeeze the juice from the half of lemon over the potatoes. Throw in the garlic cloves and the lemon wedges and give it all a really good toss together. Tuck in the rosemary stalks amongst the potatoes.
- Return the basket to the Air Fryer and cook for a further 15 minutes. Check. They should be done, but if you prefer them a little more golden, put them back on for 5 minutes.
- Pick out the woody rosemary sticks and serve the potatoes with the garlic cloves and the lemon wedges. Guests can squeeze the soft, sweet cloves of garlic out of their skins and eat it with the potatoes and the caramelized lemon.

To serve

- When serving be sure to get some of the roasted garlic cloves and lemon wedges in each portion, then while eating, smush the caramelized lemon against the potatoes, squeeze that sweet roasted garlic out of its papery skin and eat it all together. And that's your potato game changed FOREVER!

Nutrition

- Calories: 172kcal
- Carbohydrates: 28g
- Protein: 5g
- Fat: 6g
- Saturated Fat: 1g
- Sodium: 485mg
- Potassium: 817mg
- Fiber: 6g
- Sugar: 1g
- Vitamin A: 23IU
- Vitamin C: 44mg
- Calcium: 72mg
- Iron: 6mg

7. <u>**Air Fryer Broccoli**</u>

Prep Time: 5 minutes Cook Time: 15 minutes Total Time: 20 minutes

Ingredients

- 1 pound (450 grams) broccoli cut into florets
- 1 tablespoon olive oil
- ½ teaspoon salt
- ¼ teaspoon ground black pepper
- ¼ teaspoon chili flakes optional

Instructions

- Wash the broccoli head, and cut it into florets.
- In a mixing bowl, toss the broccoli florets with olive oil, salt, pepper, and chili flakes.
- Add to the Air Fryer basket, and cook at 390°F (200°C) for 15 minutes flipping at least twice while cooking.
- Serve with lemon wedges.

Nutrition

- Calories: 70kcal | Carbohydrates: 8g | Protein: 3g | Fat: 4g | Saturated Fat: 1g | Sodium: 330mg | Potassium: 358mg | Fiber: 3g | Sugar: 2g | Vitamin A: 744IU | Vitamin C: 101mg | Calcium: 53mg | Iron: 1mg

8. Air Fryer Green Beans

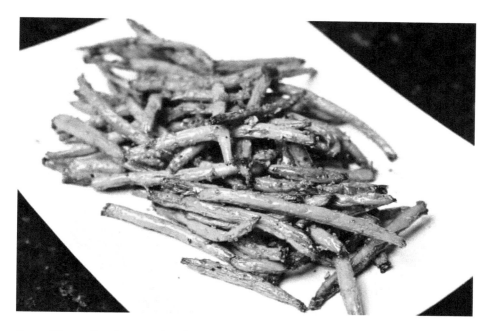

Prep Time: 5 minutes Cook Time: 10 minutes Total Time: 15 minutes

Ingredients

- 12 ounces (or 340 grams) fresh green beans, washed, trimmed, and dried
- 1 tablespoon extra virgin olive oil
- 1/2 teaspoon dried basil
- 1/2 teaspoon dried oregano
- 1/4 teaspoon garlic powder
- 1/4 teaspoon kosher salt
- Fresh lemon wedges (optional)

Instructions

- Place the green beans in a large bowl and add the oil and seasoning. Toss until well coated.
- Arrange the beans in the air fryer basket and air fry on 400F for

29

7-10 minutes (see note).
- Squeeze some fresh lemon juice over top (optional) and serve immediately.

Nutritional Facts

- Calories: 58
- Total Fat: 3.7g
- Total Carbohydrate: 6.2g
- Sugar: 2.8g
- Calcium: 35.6mg
- Sat Fat: 0.5g
- Sodium: 82.8mg
- Fiber: 2.4g
- Protein: 1.6g
- Vitamin C: 10.4mg
- Iron: 1mg

9. <u>Cauliflower</u>

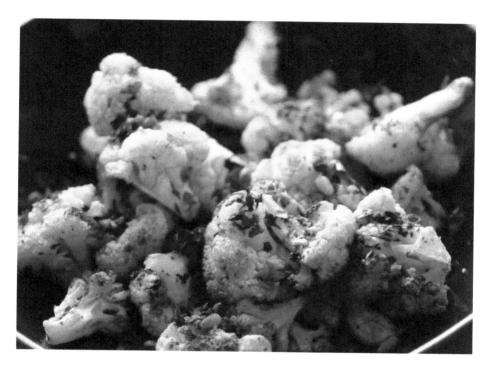

Prep Time: 8 mins

Cook Time: 12 mins

Total Time: 20 mins

Ingredients

- 1 head cauliflower
- 2 tbsp olive oil
- 1 tsp salt
- 2 tsp onion powder
- **To Top:** lime wedge and parmesan

Instructions

- Cut your cauliflower into florets.
- Toss the cauliflower in olive oil, salt, and onion salt.
- Add the cauliflower into the air fryer basket (try to have it in a single layer if possible, cook in two batches if too many overlap).
- Cook for 12-15 minutes on 375F.
- When done, serve with parmesan shaved on top and some lime squeezed on top.

Nutrition

- Serving: 4servings | Calories: 102kcal | Carbohydrates: 8g | Protein: 3g | Fat: 7g | Saturated Fat: 1g | Sodium: 626mg | Potassium: 442mg | Fiber: 3g | Sugar: 3g | Vitamin C: 70mg | Calcium: 36mg | Iron: 1mg

10. <u>Air Fryer Tater Tots</u>

Prep Time: 15 mins Cook Time: 20 mins Total Time: 35 mins

Ingredients

- 6 large potatoes or 8 medium, peeled
- 2 tbsp corn starch (cornflour)
- 1 1/2 tsp dried oregano
- 1 tsp garlic powder
- Salt

Instructions

- Preheat the air fryer to 350 F / 180C.
- Boil the potatoes till they are about half cooked and then plunge them into a cold water bath to stop the cooking process and cool them down.
- Using a box shredder, shred the cooled potatoes into a large bowl, then squeeze out any excess water.
- Add in the rest of the ingredients and combine. Then form the mixture into individual tater tots (I was able to make about 20).
- Place half of the homemade tater tots into the air fryer basket (making sure they don't touch) and cook for 18-20 minutes till golden brown. Turn the tots twice during cooking so that they brown evenly.
- Remove the tater tots and keep warm, then repeat steps to make the remaining air fryer tater tots.
- Serve your air fryer tater tots with a side of vegan ranch dressing or tomato sauce for dipping.

Nutrition

- Calories: 204kcal | Carbohydrates: 44g | Protein: 8g | Sodium: 32mg | Potassium: 1328mg | Fiber: 8g | Vitamin C: 36.4mg | Calcium: 102mg | Iron: 10.5mg

11.   **Beets (Easy Roasted Beets)**

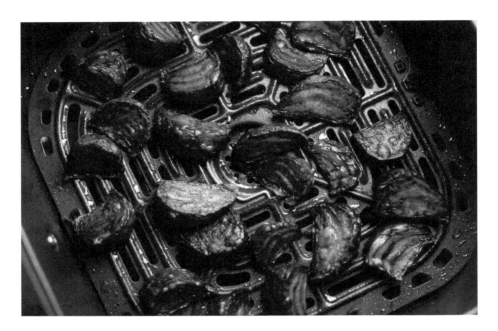

Prep Time: 10 minutes

Cook Time: 20 minutes

Total Time: 30 minutes

Ingredients

- 3 cups fresh beets, peeled and cut into 1-inch pieces (see note)
- 1 tablespoon extra virgin olive oil
- 1/2 teaspoon kosher salt
- Pinch of ground black pepper

Instructions

- Add the beets, oil, salt, and pepper to a large bowl and toss to combine.
- Place the beets in the air fryer basket and air fry on 400F for 18-

20 minutes, or until fork-tender. Stir or shake them a few times while air frying.

Nutritional Facts

- Calories: 74
- Total Fat: 3.7g
- Total Carbohydrate: 9.8g
- Sugar: 6.9g
- Calcium: 16.6mg
- Sat Fat: 0.5g
- Sodium: 234.mg
- Fiber: 2.9g
- Protein: 1.6g
- Vitamin C: 5mg
- Iron: 0.8mg

12.   Crispy Air Fryer Brussels Sprouts

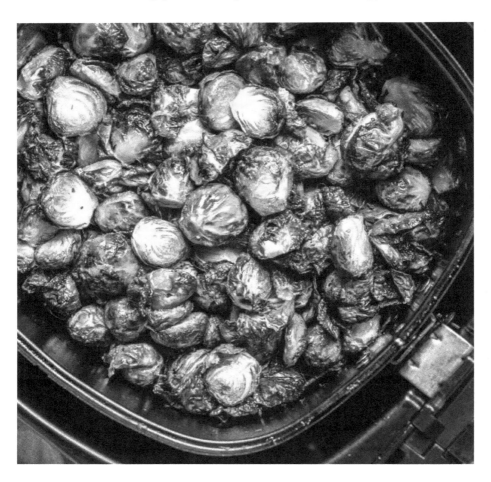

Prep Time: 5 mins

Cook Time: 10 mins

Total Time: 15 mins

Ingredients

- 340 grams Brussels sprouts
- 1-2 tbsp olive oil

- Salt, to taste
- Pepper, to taste
- Garlic powder, to taste

Instructions

- Trim and half your Brussels sprouts and lightly coat them with olive oil.
- Coat with a mixture of salt, pepper, and garlic powder.
- Place the Brussels sprouts in the air fryer at 350F for 10 minutes. Shaking the basket once or twice during the cooking time.
- Serve immediately or warm.

Nutritional Value

- Calories: 91kcal | Carbohydrates: 6g | Protein: 2g | Fat: 7g | Saturated Fat: 1g | Sodium: 300mg | Potassium: 296mg | Fiber: 1g | Sugar: 4g | Vitamin A: 196IU | Vitamin C: 20mg | Calcium: 25mg | Iron: 1mg

13. __Air-Fried Cauliflower With Almonds And Parmesan__

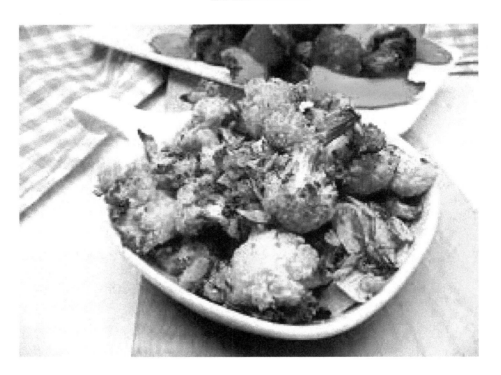

Prep: 10 mins Cook: 15 mins Total: 25 mins

Servings: 4

Ingredient

- 3 cups cauliflower florets
- 3 teaspoons vegetable oil, divided
- 1 clove garlic, minced
- ⅓ cup finely shredded Parmesan cheese
- ¼ cup chopped almonds
- ¼ cup panko bread crumbs
- ½ teaspoon dried thyme, crushed

Instructions

- Place cauliflower florets, 2 teaspoons oil, and garlic in a medium bowl; toss to coat. Place in a single layer in an air fryer basket.
- Cook in the air fryer at 360 degrees F (180 degrees C), for 10 minutes, shaking the basket halfway through.
- Return cauliflower to the bowl and toss with the remaining 1 teaspoon oil. Add Parmesan cheese, almonds, bread crumbs, and thyme; toss to coat. Return cauliflower mixture to the air fryer basket and cook until mixture is crisp and browned about 5 minutes.

Nutrition Facts

- Calories: 148; Protein 6.7g; Carbohydrates 11g; Fat 10.1g; Cholesterol 5.9mg; Sodium 157.7mg.

14. **Air Fryer Falafel**

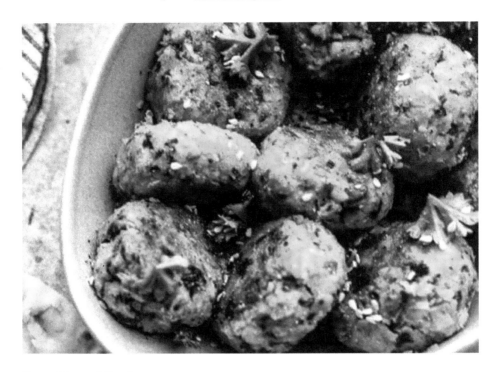

Prep Time: 20 mins

Cook: 20 mins

Additional: 1 day

Total: 1 day

Ingredient

- 1 cup dry garbanzo beans
- 1 ½ cups fresh cilantro, stems removed
- ¾ cup fresh flat-leafed parsley stems removed
- 1 small red onion, quartered
- 1 clove garlic
- 2 tablespoons chickpea flour

- 1 tablespoon ground coriander
- 1 tablespoon ground cumin
- 1 tablespoon sriracha sauce
- salt and ground black pepper to taste
- ½ teaspoon baking powder
- ¼ teaspoon baking soda
- cooking spray

Instructions

- Soak chickpeas in a large amount of cool water for 24 hours. Rub the soaked chickpeas with your fingers to help loosen and remove skins. Rinse and drain well. Spread chickpeas on a large clean dish towel to dry.
- Blend chickpeas, cilantro, parsley, onion, and garlic in a food processor until rough paste forms. Transfer mixture to a large bowl. Add chickpea flour, coriander, cumin, sriracha, salt, and pepper and mix well. Cover bowl and let the mixture rest for 1 hour.
- Preheat an air fryer to 375 degrees F (190 degrees C).
- Add baking powder and baking soda to the chickpea mixture. Mix using your hands until just combined. Form 15 equal-sized balls and press slightly to form patties. Spray falafel patties with cooking spray.
- Place 7 falafel patties in the preheated air fryer and cook for 10 minutes. Transfer cooked falafel to a plate and repeat with the remaining 8 falafel, cooking for 10 to 12 minutes.

Nutrition Facts

- Calories: 60; Protein 3.1g; Carbohydrates 9.9g; Fat 1.1g; Sodium 97.9mg.

15. <u>Air-Fried Carrots With Balsamic Glaze</u>

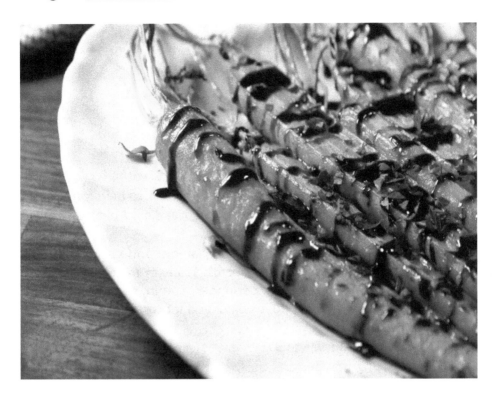

Prep Time: 10 mins

Cook Time: 10 mins

Total Time: 20 mins

Ingredient

- Olive oil for brushing
- 1 tablespoon olive oil
- 1 teaspoon honey
- ¼ teaspoon kosher salt
- ¼ teaspoon ground black pepper
- 1 pound tri-colored baby carrots

- 1 tablespoon balsamic glaze
- 1 tablespoon butter
- 2 teaspoons chopped fresh chives

Instructions

- Brush an air fryer basket with olive oil.
- Whisk together 1 tablespoon olive oil, honey, salt, and pepper in a large bowl. Add carrots and toss to coat. Place carrots in the air fryer basket in a single layer, in batches, if needed.
- Cook in the air fryer at 390 degrees F (200 degrees C), stirring once, until tender, about 10 minutes. Transfer warm cooked carrots to a large bowl, add balsamic glaze and butter and toss to coat. Sprinkle with chives and serve.

Nutrition Facts Facts

- Calories: 117; Protein 0.8g; Carbohydrates 11.9g; Fat 7.7g; Cholesterol 7.6mg; Sodium 228mg.

16.   Simple Air Fryer Brussels Sprouts

Prep Time: 5 mins

Cook Time: 30 mins

Total Time: 35 mins

Ingredient

- 1 ½ pound Brussels sprouts
- 2 tablespoons olive oil
- 1 teaspoon garlic powder
- 1 teaspoon salt
- ½ teaspoon ground black pepper

Instructions

- Preheat the air fryer to 390 degrees F (200 degrees C) for 15 minutes.
- Place Brussels sprouts, olive oil, garlic powder, salt, and pepper in a bowl and mix well. Spread evenly in the air fryer basket. Cook for 15 minutes, shaking the basket halfway through the cycle.

Nutrition Facts

- Calories: 91; Protein 3.9g; Carbohydrates 10.6g; Fat 4.8g; Sodium 416.2mg.

17. <u>Air Fryer Potato Wedges</u>

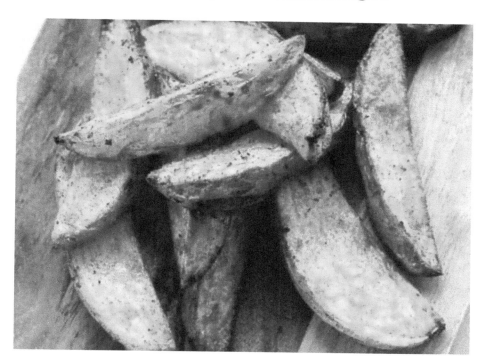

Prep Time: 5 mins

Cook Time: 30 mins

Total Time: 35 mins

Ingredient

- 2 medium Russet potatoes, cut into wedges
- 1 ½ tablespoon olive oil
- ½ teaspoon paprika
- ½ teaspoon parsley flakes
- ½ teaspoon chili powder
- ½ teaspoon sea salt
- ⅛ teaspoon ground black pepper

Instructions

- Preheat air fryer to 400 degrees F (200 degrees C).
- Place potato wedges in a large bowl. Add olive oil, paprika, parsley, chili, salt, and pepper, and mix well to combine.
- Place 8 wedges in the basket of the air fryer and cook for 10 minutes.
- Flip wedges with tongs and cook for an additional 5 minutes. Repeat with the remaining 8 wedges.

Nutrition Facts

- Calories: 129; Protein 2.3g; Carbohydrates 19g; Fat 5.3g; Sodium 230.2mg.

18.   Air-Fryer Roasted Veggies

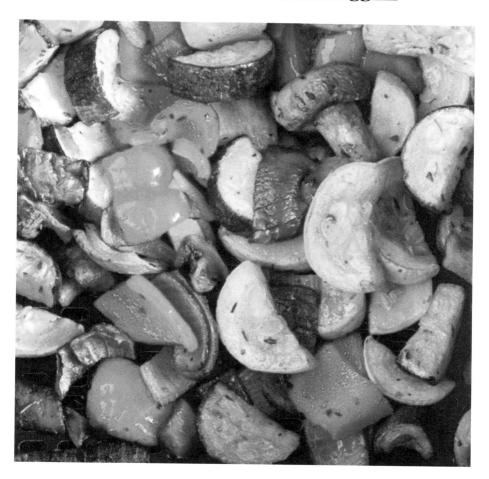

Prep Time: 20 mins

Cook Time: 10 mins

Total Time: 30 mins

Ingredient

- ½ cup diced zucchini
- ½ cup diced summer squash

- ½ cup diced mushrooms
- ½ cup diced cauliflower
- ½ cup diced asparagus
- ½ cup diced sweet red pepper
- 2 teaspoons vegetable oil
- ¼ teaspoon salt
- ¼ teaspoon ground black pepper
- 1/4 teaspoon seasoning, or more to taste

Instructions

- Preheat the air fryer to 360 degrees F (180 degrees C).
- Add vegetables, oil, salt, pepper, and desired seasoning to a bowl. Toss to coat; arrange in the fryer basket.
- Cook vegetables for 10 minutes, stirring after 5 minutes.

Nutrition Facts Facts

- Calories:37; Protein 1.4g; Carbohydrates 3.4g; Fat 2.4g; Sodium 152.2mg.

19. **Air Fryer Roasted Asparagus**

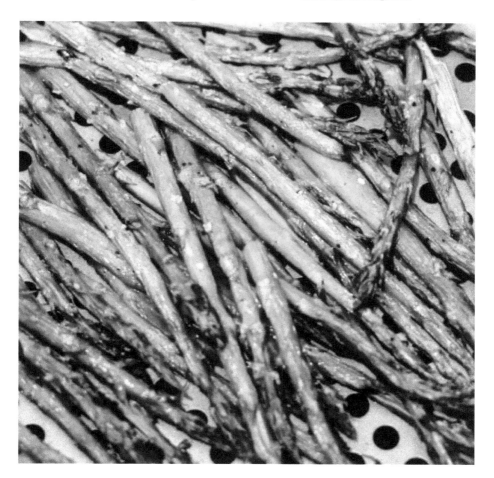

Prep Time: 10 mins

Cook Time: 10 mins

Total Time: 20 mins

Ingredient

- 1 bunch fresh asparagus, trimmed
- Avocado oil cooking spray

- ½ teaspoon garlic powder
- ½ teaspoon himalayan pink salt
- ¼ teaspoon ground multi-colored peppercorns
- ¼ teaspoon red pepper flakes
- ¼ cup freshly grated parmesan cheese

Instructions

- Preheat the air fryer to 375 degrees F (190 degrees C). Line the basket with parchment paper.
- Place asparagus spears in the air fryer basket and mist with avocado oil. Sprinkle with garlic powder, pink Himalayan salt, pepper, and red pepper flakes. Top with Parmesan cheese.
- Air fry until asparagus spears start to char, 7 to 9 minutes.

Nutrition Facts

- Calories: 94; Protein 9g; Carbohydrates 10.1g; Fat 3.3g; Cholesterol 8.8mg; Sodium 739.2mg.

20. <u>Air Fryer Sweet And Spicy Roasted Carrots</u>

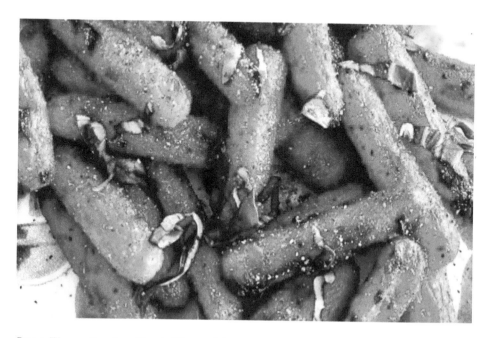

Prep Time: 5 mins Cook Time: 20 mins Total: 25 mins

Ingredient

- 1 serving cooking spray
- 1 tablespoon butter, melted
- 1 tablespoon hot honey (such as Mike's Hot Honey®)
- 1 teaspoon grated orange zest
- ½ teaspoon ground cardamom
- ½ pound baby carrots
- 1 tablespoon freshly squeezed orange juice
- 1 pinch salt and ground black pepper to taste

Instructions

- Preheat an air fryer to 400 degrees F (200 degrees C). Spray the

basket with nonstick cooking spray.
- Combine butter, honey, orange zest, and cardamom in a bowl. Remove 1 tablespoon of the sauce to a separate bowl and set aside. Add carrots to the remaining sauce and toss until all are well coated. Transfer carrots to the air fryer basket.
- Air fry until carrots are roasted and fork-tender, tossing every 7 minutes, for 15 to 22 minutes. Mix orange juice with reserved honey-butter sauce. Toss with carrots until well combined. Season with salt and pepper.

Nutrition Facts

Calories: 129; Protein 0.9g; Carbohydrates 19.3g; Fat 6.1g; Cholesterol 15.3mg; Sodium 206.4mg.

21.   Air Fryer One-Bite Roasted Potatoes

Prep Time: 5 mins

Cook Time: 10 mins

Total Time: 15 mins

Ingredient

- ½ Pound mini potatoes
- 2 teaspoons extra-virgin olive oil
- 2 teaspoons dry italian-style salad dressing mix
- Salt and ground black pepper to taste

Instructions

- Preheat the air fryer to 400 degrees F (200 degrees C).
- Wash and dry potatoes. Trim edges to make a flat surface on both ends.
- Combine extra-virgin olive oil and salad dressing mix in a large bowl. Add potatoes and toss until potatoes are well coated. Place in a single layer into the air fryer basket. Cook in batches if necessary.
- Air fry until potatoes are golden brown, 5 to 7 minutes. Flip potatoes and air fry for an additional 2 to 3 minutes. Season with salt and pepper.

Nutrition Facts

- Calories: 132; Protein 2.3g; Carbohydrates 20.3g; Fat 4.8g; Sodium 166.8mg.

22. **Air Fryer Cauliflower Tots**

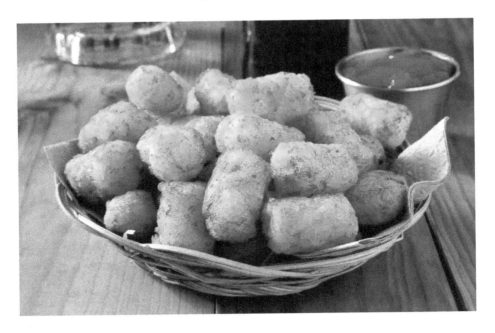

Prep Time: 5 mins

Cook Time: 10 mins

Total Time: 15 mins

Ingredient

- 1 serving nonstick cooking spray
- 1 (16 ounces) package frozen cauliflower tots (such as Green Giant® Cauliflower Veggie Tots)

Instructions

- Preheat air fryer to 400 degrees F (200 degrees C). Spray the air fryer basket with nonstick cooking spray.
- Place as many cauliflower tots in the basket as you can, making sure they do not touch, cooking in batches if necessary.

- Cook in the preheated air fryer for 6 minutes. Pull the basket out, turn tots over, and cook until browned and cooked through, about 3 minutes more.

Nutrition Facts Facts

- Calories: 147; Protein 2.7g; Carbohydrates 20g; Fat 6.1g; Sodium 493.6mg.

23. <u>Sweet Potato Tots</u>

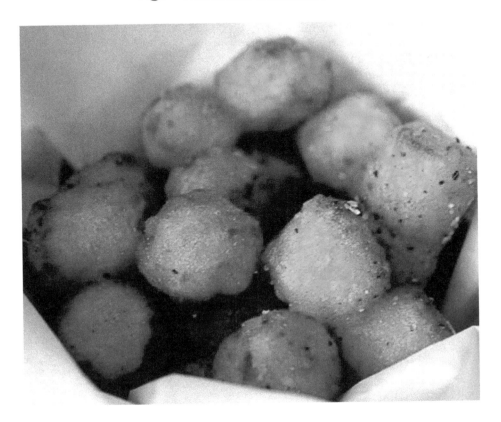

Prep Time: 15 mins

Cook Time: 35 mins

Additional Time: 10 mins

Total Time: 1 hr

Ingredient

- 2 sweet potatoes, peeled
- ½ teaspoon cajun seasoning
- Olive oil cooking spray

- Sea salt to taste

Instructions

- Bring a pot of water to a boil and add sweet potatoes. Boil until potatoes can be pierced with a fork but are still firm for about 15 minutes. Do not over-boil, or they will be messy to grate. Drain and let cool.
- Grate sweet potatoes into a bowl using a box grater. Carefully mix in Cajun seasoning. Form mixture into tot-shaped cylinders.
- Spray the air fryer basket with olive oil spray. Place tots in the basket in a single row without touching each other or the sides of the basket. Spray tots with olive oil spray and sprinkle with sea salt.
- Heat air fryer to 400 degrees F (200 degrees C) and cook tots for 8 minutes. Turn, spray with more olive oil spray, and sprinkle with more sea salt. Cook for 8 minutes more.

Nutrition Facts

- Calories: 21; Protein 0.4g; Carbohydrates 4.8g; Sodium 36.2mg.

24. **Air Fryer Fried Green Tomatoes**

Prep Time: 15 mins

Cook Time: 20 mins

Total Time: 35 mins

Ingredient

- 2 green tomatoes, cut into 1/4-inch slices
- Salt and freshly ground black pepper to taste
- ⅓ cup all-purpose flour
- ½ cup buttermilk
- 2 eggs, lightly beaten
- 1 cup plain panko bread crumbs
- 1 cup yellow cornmeal
- 1 teaspoon garlic powder
- ½ teaspoon paprika
- 1 tablespoon olive oil, or as needed

Instructions

- Season tomato slices with salt and pepper.
- Set up a breading station in 3 shallow dishes: pour flour into the first dish; stir together buttermilk and eggs in the second dish; and mix breadcrumbs, cornmeal, garlic powder, and paprika in the third dish.
- Dredge tomato slices in flour, shaking off the excess. Dip tomatoes into the egg mixture, and then into the bread crumb mixture, making sure to coat both sides.
- Preheat the air fryer to 400 degrees F (200 degrees C). Brush the fryer basket with olive oil. Place breaded tomato slices in the fryer basket, making sure they do not touch each other; cook in batches if necessary. Brush the tops of tomatoes with olive oil.

- Cook for 12 minutes, then flip the tomatoes and brush again with olive oil. Cook until crisp and golden brown, 3 to 5 minutes more. Remove tomatoes to a paper towel-lined rack to keep crisp. Repeat with the remaining tomatoes.

Nutrition Facts

- Calories: 219; Protein 7.6g; Carbohydrates 39.6g; Fat 5.3g; Cholesterol 62.8mg; Sodium 165.9mg.

25.   <u>Air Fryer Latkes</u>

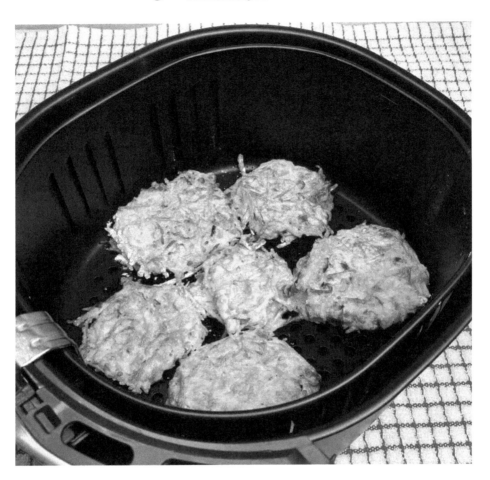

Prep Time: 20 mins

Cook Time: 20 mins

Total Time: 40 mins

Ingredient

- 1 (16 ounces) package frozen shredded hash brown potatoes, thawed

- ½ cup shredded onion
- 1 egg
- Kosher salt and ground black pepper to taste
- 2 tablespoons matzo meal
- Avocado oil cooking spray

Instructions

- Preheat an air fryer to 375 degrees F (190 degrees C) according to the manufacturer's instructions. Layout a sheet of parchment or waxed paper.
- Place thawed potatoes and shredded onion on several layers of paper towels. Cover with more paper towels and press to squeeze out most of the liquid.
- Whisk together egg, salt, and pepper in a large bowl. Stir in potatoes and onion with a fork. Sprinkle matzo meal on top and stir until ingredients are evenly distributed. Use your hands to form the mixture into ten 3- to 4-inch wide patties. Place patties on the parchment or waxed paper.
- Spray the air fryer basket with cooking spray. Carefully place half of the patties in the basket and spray generously with cooking spray.
- Air-fry until crispy and dark golden brown on the outside, 10 to 12 minutes. (Check for doneness at 8 minutes if you prefer a softer latke.) Remove latkes to a plate. Repeat with remaining patties, spraying them with cooking spray before cooking.

Nutrition Facts

- Calories: 97; Protein 3.3g; Carbohydrates 18.6g; Fat 6.5g; Cholesterol 32.7mg; Sodium 121.3mg.

26. Truffle Fries

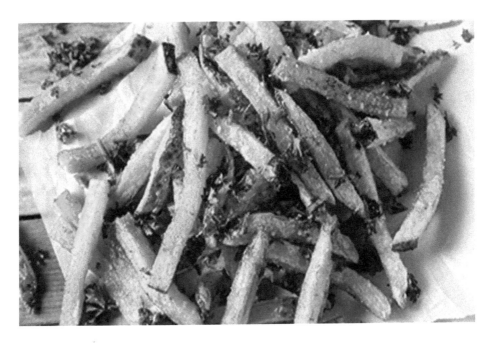

Prep Time: 10 mins

Cook Time: 20 mins

Additional Time: 30 mins

Total Time: 1 hr

Ingredient

- 1 ¾ pounds russet potatoes, peeled and cut into fries
- 2 tablespoons truffle-infused olive oil
- ½ teaspoon paprika
- 1 tablespoon grated Parmesan cheese
- 2 teaspoons chopped fresh parsley
- 1 teaspoon black truffle sea salt

Instructions

- Place fries in a bowl. Cover with water and let soak for 30 minutes. Drain and pat dry.
- Preheat the air fryer to 400 degrees F (200 degrees C) according to the manufacturer's **Instructions**.
- Place drained fries into a large bowl. Add truffle olive oil and paprika; stir until evenly combined. Transfer fries to the air fryer basket.
- Air fry for 20 minutes, shaking every 5 minutes. Transfer fries to a bowl. Add Parmesan cheese, parsley, and truffle salt. Toss to coat.

Nutrition Facts

- Calories: 226; Protein 4.8g; Carbohydrates 36.1g; Fat 7.6g; Cholesterol 1.1mg; Sodium 552mg.

27. **Spaghetti Squash**

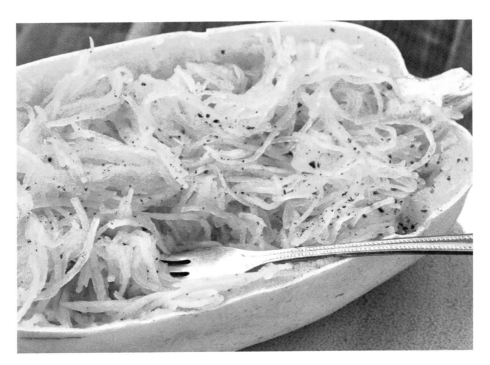

Prep Time: 5 mins

Cook Time: 25 mins

Total Time: 30 mins

Ingredient

- 1 (3 pounds) spaghetti squash
- 1 teaspoon olive oil
- ¼ teaspoon sea salt
- ⅛ teaspoon ground black pepper
- ⅛ teaspoon smoked paprika

Instructions

- Using a sharp knife, make a dotted line lengthwise around the entire squash. Place whole squash in the microwave and cook on full power for 5 minutes. Transfer to a cutting board and cut the squash in half lengthwise, using the dotted line as a guide. Wrap one half in plastic wrap and refrigerate for another use.
- Spoon pulp and seeds out of the remaining half and discard. Brush olive oil over all of the flesh and sprinkle with salt, pepper, and paprika.
- Preheat an air fryer to 360 degrees F (180 degrees C). Place spaghetti squash half skin-side-down in the basket. Cook for 20 minutes.
- Transfer to a dish and fluff with a fork to create 'noodles'.

Nutrition Facts

Calories: 223; Protein 4.4g; Carbohydrates 47.2g; Fat 6.3g; Sodium 335.9mg.

28. Air Fryer Roasted Brussels Sprouts With Maple-Mustard Mayo

Prep Time: 5 mins Cook Time: 10 mins Total Time: 15 mins

Ingredient

- 2 tablespoons maple syrup, divided
- 1 tablespoon olive oil
- ¼ teaspoon kosher salt
- ¼ teaspoon ground black pepper
- 1 pound Brussels sprouts, trimmed and halved
- ⅓ cup mayonnaise
- 1 tablespoon stone-ground mustard

Instructions

- Preheat the air fryer to 400 degrees F (200 degrees C).
- Whisk together 1 tablespoon maple syrup, olive oil, salt, and pepper in a large bowl. Add Brussels sprouts and toss to coat. Arrange Brussels sprouts in a single layer in an air fryer basket without overcrowding; work in batches, if necessary. Cook for 4 minutes. Shake basket and cook until sprouts are deep golden brown and tender, 4 to 6 minutes more.
- Meanwhile, whisk together mayonnaise, remaining 1 tablespoon maple syrup, and mustard in a small bowl. Toss sprouts in some of the sauce mixtures and/or serve as a dipping sauce.

Nutrition Facts

Calories: 240; Protein 4g; Carbohydrates 18.3g; Fat 18.3g; Cholesterol 7mg; Sodium 298mg.

29. <u>Peri Peri Fries</u>

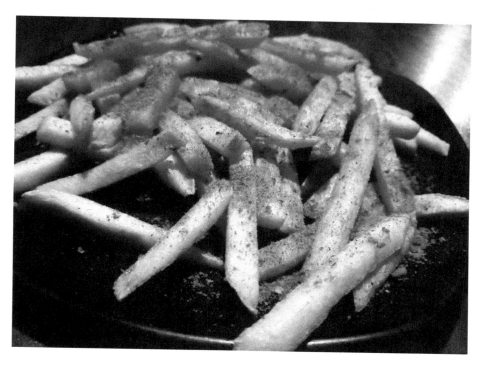

Prep Time: 10 mins

Cook Time: 25 mins

Additional Time: 15 mins

Total Time: 50 mins

Ingredient

- 2 pounds russet potatoes
- ¼ teaspoon smoked paprika
- ¼ teaspoon chile powder
- ¼ teaspoon garlic granules
- ⅛ teaspoon ground white pepper
- ½ teaspoon salt

67

- 2 tablespoons grapeseed oil

Instructions

- Peel and cut potatoes into 3/8-inch slices. Place into a bowl of water for 15 minutes to remove most of the starch. Transfer onto a clean kitchen towel and dry.
- Preheat the air fryer to 350 degrees F (180 degrees C) for 5 minutes.
- Mix paprika, chile powder, garlic. white pepper, and salt together in a small bowl.
- Place the potatoes into a medium bowl and add grapeseed oil; mix well. Pour into the air fryer basket.
- Air fry for 10 minutes, shaking occasionally. Increase the temperature to 400 degrees F (200 degrees C) and air fry until golden brown, 12 to 15 more minutes.
- Pour fries into a bowl, sprinkle with the seasoning mix, and shake the bowl to ensure fries are evenly covered. Taste and adjust salt, if necessary. Serve immediately.

Nutrition Facts

- Calories: 237; Protein 4.7g; Carbohydrates 40g; Fat 7.1g; Sodium 304.4mg.

30. Air Fryer Fish And Chips

Prep Time: 20 mins

Cook Time: 30 mins

Additional Time: 1 hr 10 mins

Total Time: 2 hrs

Ingredients

Chips:

- 1 russet potato
- 2 teaspoons vegetable oil
- 1 pinch salt and ground black pepper to taste

Fish:

- ¾ cup all-purpose flour
- 2 tablespoons cornstarch
- ½ teaspoon salt
- ½ teaspoon garlic powder
- ¼ teaspoon baking soda
- ¼ teaspoon baking powder
- ¾ cup malt beer
- 4 (3 ounces) fillets cod fillets

Instructions

- Peel the russet potato and cut it into 12 wedges. Pour 3 cups water into a medium bowl and submerge potato wedges for 15 minutes. Drain off water and replace it with fresh water. Soak wedges for 15 more minutes.
- Meanwhile, mix flour, cornstarch, salt, garlic powder, baking soda, and baking powder in a bowl. Pour in 1/2 cup malt beer

and stir to combine. If batter seems too thick, add remaining beer 1 tablespoon at a time.

- Place cod fillets on a rimmed baking sheet lined with a drip rack. Spoon 1/2 of the batter over the fillets. Place rack in the freezer to allow the batter to solidify, about 35 minutes. Flip fillets over and coat the remaining side with the batter. Return to the freezer for an additional 35 minutes.
- Preheat the air fryer to 400 degrees F (200 degrees C) for 8 minutes.
- Cook frozen fish fillets for 15 minutes, flipping at the halfway point.
- Meanwhile, drain off water from potato wedges and blot dry with a paper towel. Toss with oil, salt, and pepper. Air fry for 15 minutes.

Nutrition Facts

- Calories: 465; Protein 37.5g; Carbohydrates 62.3g; Fat 6.2g; Cholesterol 62.3mg; Sodium 1006mg.

31. "Everything" Seasoning Air Fryer Asparagus

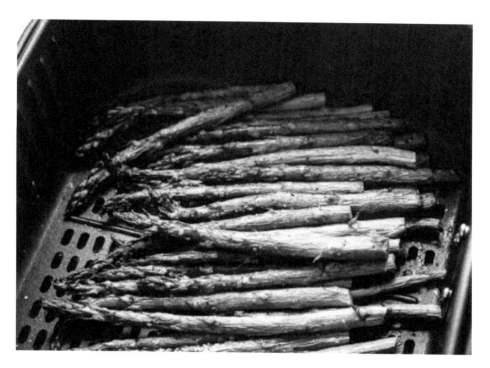

Prep Time: 5 mins

Cook Time: 5 mins

Total Time: 10 mins

Ingredient

- 1 pound thin asparagus
- 1 tablespoon olive oil
- 1 tablespoon everything bagel seasoning
- 1 pinch salt to taste
- 4 wedge (blank)s lemon wedges

Instructions

- Rinse and trim asparagus, cutting off any woody ends. Place asparagus on a plate and drizzle with olive oil. Toss with bagel seasoning until evenly combined. Place asparagus in the air fryer basket in a single layer. Work in batches if needed.
- Heat the air fryer to 390 degrees F (200 degrees C).
- Air fry until slightly soft, tossing with tongs halfway through, 5 to 6 minutes. Taste and season with salt if needed. Serve with lemon wedges.

Nutrition Facts

- Calories: 70; Protein 2.7g; Carbohydrates 5.8g; Fat 3.6g; Sodium 281.5mg.

32. Tajin Sweet Potato Fries

Prep Time: 10 mins Cook Time: 10 mins Total Time: 20 mins

Ingredient

- Cooking spray
- 2 medium sweet potatoes, cut into 1/2-inch-thick fries
- 3 teaspoons avocado oil
- 1 ½ teaspoon chili-lime seasoning (such as tajin)

Dipping Sauce:

- ¼ cup mayonnaise
- 1 tablespoon freshly squeezed lime juice
- 1 teaspoon chili-lime seasoning (such as Tajin®)
- 4 lime wedges

Instructions

- Preheat the air fryer to 400 degrees F (200 degrees C) for 5 minutes. Lightly spray the fryer basket with cooking spray.
- Place sweet potato fries in a large bowl, drizzle with avocado oil, and stir. Sprinkle with 1 1/2 teaspoons chili-lime seasoning and toss well. Transfer to the air fryer basket, working in batches if necessary.
- Cook sweet potato fries until brown and crispy, 8 to 9 minutes, shaking and turning the fries after 4 minutes.
- While sweet potatoes are cooking, whisk together mayonnaise, lime juice, and chili-lime seasoning for the dipping sauce in a small bowl. Serve sweet potato fries with dipping sauce and lime wedges.

Nutrition Facts

- Calories: 233; Protein 2g; Carbohydrates 24.1g; Fat 14.8g; Cholesterol 5.2mg; Sodium 390.1mg.

33. **Fingerling Potatoes**

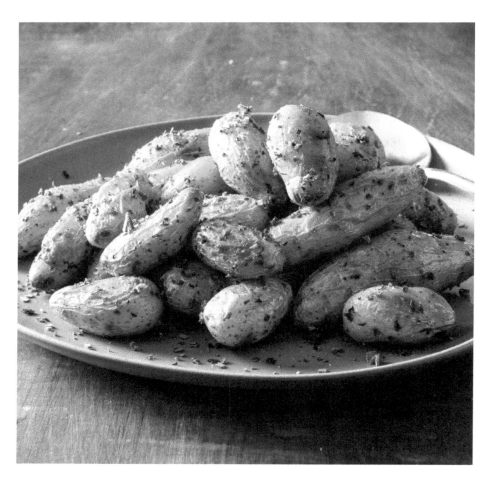

Prep Time: 10 mins

Cook Time: 15 mins

Total Time: 25 mins

Ingredient

- 1 pound fingerling potatoes, halved lengthwise
- 1 tablespoon olive oil

- ½ teaspoon ground paprika
- ½ teaspoon parsley flakes
- ½ teaspoon garlic powder
- Salt and ground black pepper to taste

Instructions

- Preheat an air fryer to 400 degrees F (200 degrees C).
- Place potato halves in a large bowl. Add olive oil, paprika, parsley, garlic powder, salt, and pepper and stir until evenly coated.
- Place potatoes in the basket of the preheated air fryer and cook for 10 minutes. Stir and cook until desired crispness is reached, about 5 more minutes.

Nutrition Facts

- Calories: 120; Protein 2.4g; Carbohydrates 20.3g; Fat 3.5g; Sodium 46.5mg.

34. <u>Sweet and Spicy Air Fried Sweet Potatoes</u>

Prep Time: 10 mins

Cook Time: 15 mins

Total Time: 25 mins

Ingredient

- 1 large sweet potato, cut into 1/2-inch pieces
- 1 tablespoon olive oil
- 1 tablespoon packed light brown sugar
- ¼ teaspoon sea salt
- ¼ teaspoon chili powder
- ¼ teaspoon ground paprika
- ¼ teaspoon cayenne pepper
- ⅛ teaspoon onion powder
- Ground black pepper to taste

Instructions

- Preheat an air fryer to 400 degrees F (200 degrees C) according to the manufacturer's **Instructions**.
- Place sweet potato in a large bowl. Drizzle with olive oil, then add brown sugar, salt, chili powder, paprika, cayenne pepper, onion powder, and pepper. Stir until potatoes are evenly coated and spread out onto the air fryer rack.
- Cook on the upper rack of the preheated air fryer until browned and crispy, 15 to 20 minutes.

Nutrition Facts

- Calories: 189; Protein 2.5g; Carbohydrates 35.3g; Fat 4.7g; Sodium 233.6mg.

35. Rosemary Potato Wedges

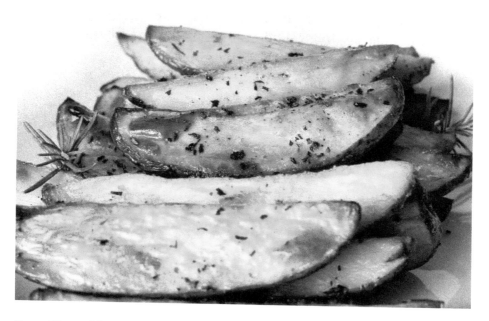

Prep Time: 10 mins

Cook Time: 20 mins

Total Time: 30 mins

Ingredient

- 2 russet potatoes, sliced into 12 wedges each with skin on
- 1 tablespoon extra-virgin olive oil
- 2 teaspoons seasoned salt
- 1 tablespoon finely chopped fresh rosemary

Instructions

- Preheat an air fryer to 380 degrees F (190 degrees C).
- Place potatoes in a large bowl and toss with olive oil. Sprinkle with seasoned salt and rosemary and toss to combine.

- Place potatoes in an even layer in a fryer basket once the air fryer is hot; you may need to cook them in batches.
- Air fry potatoes for 10 minutes, then flip wedges with tongs. Continue air frying until potato wedges reach the desired doneness, about 10 minutes more.

Nutrition Facts

- Calories: 115; Protein 2.2g; Carbohydrates 19.2g; Fat 3.5g; Sodium 465.3mg.

36. Air Fryer Roasted Cauliflower

Prep Time: 10 mins

Cook Time: 15 mins

Total Time: 25 mins

Ingredient

- 3 cloves garlic
- 1 tablespoon peanut oil
- ½ teaspoon salt
- ½ teaspoon smoked paprika
- 4 cups cauliflower florets

Instructions

- Preheat an air fryer to 400 degrees F (200 degrees C).
- Cut garlic in half and smash with the blade of a knife. Place in a bowl with oil, salt, and paprika. Add cauliflower and turn to coat.
- Place the coated cauliflower in the bowl of the air fryer and cook to desired crispiness, shaking every 5 minutes, about 15 minutes total.

Nutrition Facts

- Calories: 118; Protein 4.3g; Carbohydrates 12.4g; Fat 7g; Sodium 642.3mg.

37.   Air-Fried Ratatouille, Italian-Style

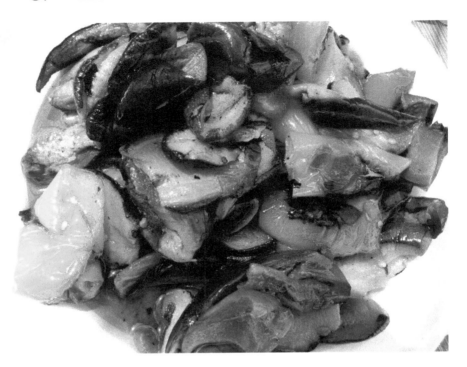

Prep Time: 25 mins

Cook Time: 25 mins

Additional Time: 5 mins

Total Time: 55 mins

Ingredient

- ½ small eggplant, cut into cubes
- 1 zucchini, cut into cubes
- 1 medium tomato, cut into cubes
- ½ large yellow bell pepper, cut into cubes
- ½ large red bell pepper, cut into cubes
- ½ onion, cut into cubes

- 1 fresh cayenne pepper, diced
- 5 sprigs fresh basil, stemmed and chopped
- 2 sprigs of fresh oregano, stemmed and chopped
- 1 clove garlic, crushed
- salt and ground black pepper to taste
- 1 tablespoon olive oil
- 1 tablespoon white wine
- 1 teaspoon vinegar

Instructions

- Preheat an air fryer to 400 degrees F (200 degrees C).
- Place eggplant, zucchini, tomato, bell peppers, and onion in a bowl. Add cayenne pepper, basil, oregano, garlic, salt, and pepper. Mix well to distribute everything evenly. Drizzle in oil, wine, and vinegar, mixing to coat all the vegetables.
- Pour vegetable mixture into a baking dish and insert it into the basket of the air fryer. Cook for 8 minutes. Stir; cook for another 8 minutes. Stir again and continue cooking until tender, stirring every 5 minutes, 10 to 15 minutes more. Turn off the air fryer, leaving the dish inside. Let rest for 5 minutes before serving.

Nutritional Value

- Calories: 79; Protein 2.1g; Carbohydrates 10.2g; Fat 3.8g; Sodium 47.6mg.

38. <u>Air Fryer Spicy Green Beans</u>

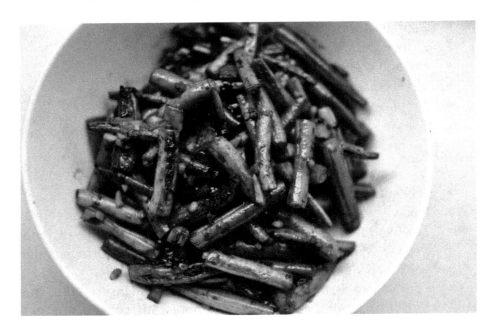

Prep Time: 10 mins

Cook Time: 25 mins

Additional Time: 5 mins

Total Time: 40 mins

Ingredient

- 12 ounces fresh green beans, trimmed
- 1 tablespoon sesame oil
- 1 teaspoon soy sauce
- 1 teaspoon rice wine vinegar
- 1 clove garlic, minced
- ½ teaspoon red pepper flakes

Instructions

- Preheat an air fryer to 400 degrees F (200 degrees C).
- Place green beans in a bowl. Whisk together sesame oil, soy sauce, rice wine vinegar, garlic, and red pepper flakes in a separate bowl and pour over green beans. Toss to coat and let marinate for 5 minutes.
- Place half the green beans in the air fryer basket. Cook 12 minutes, shaking the basket halfway through cooking time. Repeat with remaining green beans.

Nutrition Facts

- Calories: 60; Protein 1.7g; Carbohydrates 6.6g; Fat 3.6g; Sodium 80mg.

39. <u>Chinese Five-Spice Air Fryer Butternut Squash Fries</u>

Prep Time: 15 mins

Cook Time: 15 mins

Total Time: 30 mins

Ingredient

- 1 large butternut squash, peeled and cut into "fries"
- 2 tablespoons olive oil
- 1 tablespoon Chinese five-spice powder
- 1 tablespoon minced garlic
- 2 teaspoons sea salt
- 2 teaspoons black pepper

Instructions

- Preheat the air fryer to 400 degrees F (200 degrees C).
- Place cut the squash in a large bowl. Add oil, five-spice powder, garlic, salt, and black pepper, and toss to coat.
- Cook butternut squash fries in the preheated air fryer, shaking every 5 minutes, until crisp, 15 to 20 minutes total. Remove fries and season with additional sea salt.

Nutrition Facts

- Calories: 150; Protein 2.5g; Carbohydrates 28.5g; Fat 4.9g; Sodium 596.4mg.

40.   <u>Brussels Sprouts</u>

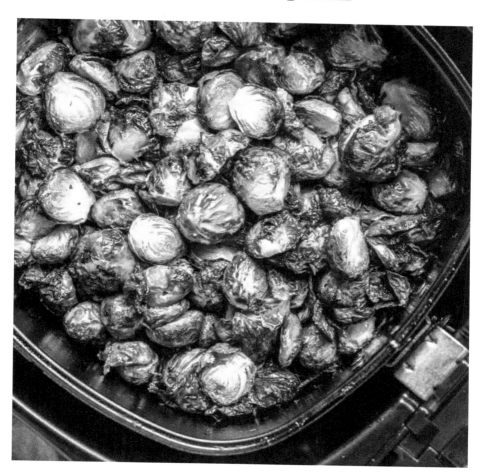

Prep Time: 5 mins

Cook Time: 10 mins

Total Time: 15 mins

Ingredient

- 1 teaspoon avocado oil
- ½ teaspoon salt

- ½ teaspoon ground black pepper
- 10 ounces Brussels sprouts, trimmed and halved lengthwise
- 1 teaspoon balsamic vinegar
- 2 teaspoons crumbled cooked bacon (optional)

Instructions

- Preheat an air fryer to 350 degrees F (175 degrees C).
- Combine oil, salt, and pepper in a bowl and mix well. Add Brussels sprouts and turn to coat.
- Air fry for 5 minutes, shake the sprouts and cook for an additional 5 minutes.
- Transfer sprouts to a serving dish and sprinkles with balsamic vinegar; turn to coat. Sprinkle with bacon.

Nutrition Facts

- Calories: 94; Protein 5.8g; Carbohydrates 13.3g; Fat 3.4g; Cholesterol 1.7mg; Sodium 690.6mg.

41.   <u>**Root Vegetables With Vegan Aioli**</u>

Prep Time: 30 mins

Cook Time: 30 mins

Total Time: 1 hr

Ingredients

Garlic Aioli:

- ½ cup vegan mayonnaise (such as Vegenaise)
- 1 clove garlic, minced
- ½ teaspoon fresh lemon juice
- Salt and ground black pepper to taste

Root Vegetables:

- 4 tablespoons extra virgin olive oil
- 1 tablespoon minced fresh rosemary
- 3 cloves garlic, finely minced
- 1 teaspoon kosher salt, or to taste
- ½ teaspoon ground black pepper, or to taste
- 1 pound parsnips, peeled and cut vertically into uniform pieces
- 1 pound baby red potatoes, cut lengthwise into 4 or 6 pieces
- ½ pound baby carrots split lengthwise
- ½ red onion cut lengthwise into 1/2-inch slices
- ½ teaspoon grated lemon zest, or to taste (Optional)

Instructions

- Combine mayonnaise, garlic, lemon juice, salt, and pepper in a small bowl for the garlic aioli; place in the refrigerator until ready to serve.
- Preheat the air fryer to 400 degrees F (200 degrees C) if your air fryer manufacturer recommends preheating.

- Combine olive oil, rosemary, garlic, salt, and pepper in a small bowl; set aside to allow the flavors to mingle. Combine parsnips, potatoes, carrots, and onion in a large bowl. Add olive oil-rosemary mixture and stir until vegetables are evenly coated. Place a portion of vegetables in a single layer in the basket of the air fryer, then add a rack and another layer of vegetables.
- Air fry for 15 minutes.
- When the timer sounds, you may plate the veggies and keep warm, or continue cooking in 5-minute intervals until the vegetables reach desired doneness and browning.
- Place remaining vegetables in the bottom of the air fryer basket and air fry for 15 minutes, checking for doneness, as needed. Use the rack again, if you have more vegetables then fit in a single layer. When all the vegetables have cooked, serve with garlic aioli and garnish with lemon zest.

Nutrition Facts

calories; protein 2.2g; carbohydrates 25.5g; fat 13.8g; sodium 338.3mg.

42. <u>Air Fryer Roasted Broccoli And Cauliflower</u>

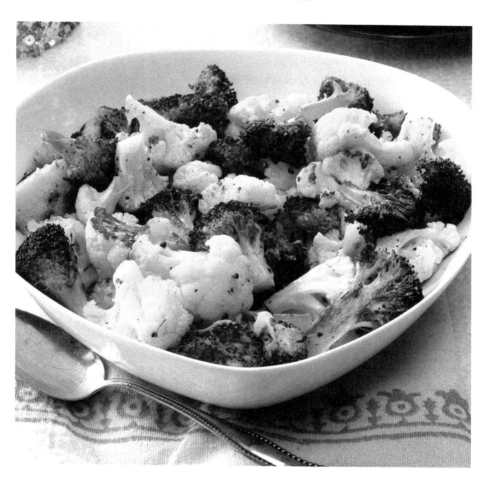

Prep Time: 10 mins

Cook Time: 15 mins

Total Time: 25 mins

Ingredient

- 3 cups broccoli florets
- 3 cups cauliflower florets
- 2 tablespoons olive oil
- ½ teaspoon garlic powder
- ¼ teaspoon sea salt
- ¼ teaspoon paprika
- ⅛ teaspoon ground black pepper

Instructions

- Heat an air fryer to 400 degrees F (200 degrees C) following the manufacturer's instructions.
- Place broccoli florets in a large, microwave-safe bowl. Cook in the microwave on high power for 3 minutes. Drain any accumulated liquid.
- Add cauliflower, olive oil, garlic powder, sea salt, paprika, and black pepper to the bowl with the broccoli. Mix well to combine. Pour mixture into the air fryer basket. Cook for 12 minutes, tossing vegetables halfway through cooking time for even browning.

Nutrition Facts

Calories: 68; Protein 2.3g; Carbohydrates 5.8g; Fat 4.7g; Sodium 103.1mg.

CPSIA information can be obtained
at www.ICGtesting.com
Printed in the USA
BVHW050324080521
606757BV00010B/1629